ERLINDA TULIOC

Women's Beginners Fitness Sense After 50

A Practical Guide to Your Fitness Journey Success

First edition

This book was professionally typeset on Reedsy.
Find out more at reedsy.com

Tim, your light shines on within my heart!

Aging is an extraordinary process whereby you become the person you always should have been.

DAVID BOWIE

Contents

One

INTRODUCTION

꧁꧂

AGING WISE

Congratulations on investing in your health and fitness. I'm so excited to be able to share my insights on fitness sense for women, fifty years of age and beyond. My name is Erlinda Tulioc, I'm a mother of two beautiful grown children. I worked a full-time job, and made time for my husband and children, but had very little free time for myself. It was not unusual for me to be working over 40 hours per week, taking my children to their various practices, then coming home preparing dinner, making sure homework was checked and completed, and endeavoring to spend quality time with my husband.

This left very little free time for me. As you know there are only 24 hours in a day so my consistent pursuit of fitness took a holiday. This holiday took a number of years. My attempts to restart a consistent fitness program were definitely a challenge. As the years flew by, I noticed I slowly lost my endurance to be able to walk up and down stairs without getting winded. I found the size of my clothes getting bigger, my weight blossoming, my blood pressure rising, and on the cusp of pre-diabetes. My health became a concern and I could see my existence on this earth slowly diminishing. You see, I have a degree in Human Performance (Physical Education) with a minor in Health. To find myself in this situation was a bit embarrassing yet, it served as a sobering wake-up call to get back on a reasonable fitness journey.

Now that I'm a bit older and on many counts, a bit wiser, I realize the importance of being fit. Furthermore, I have a greater appreciation of how my fitness level enhances my ability to engage in many different types of activities that require active involvement. I prefer to do it for myself rather than having others do it for me. I want to remain a participant in life instead of life passing me by. What about you?

Women, as we get older our metabolism slows down, so it's easier to gain weight. Our balance can be easily compromised so you may find yourself tripping on nonexistent level changes on the rug or floor. Our strength becomes weaker so opening those pesky jelly jars seems nearly impossible. Picking up or trying to keep up with the energetic kids or grandkids is becoming more difficult. Negotiating a walk from the concrete sidewalk to uneven grass, or even to open sand seemed like a major obstacle difficult to overcome. However take heart, that investing in your fitness can reverse many of these concerns.

I created this book as a practical common sense fitness guide for women to help put perspective on their fitness pursuits. I look at the importance of having a positive mindset, recognizing our different body types, diets, and quality of sleep, and finding the "right" fitness intensity to meet your fitness goal and exercises.

Many of the criteria used to define fitness for women are based on research done on men. The mistaken belief was that women were just smaller men so therefore, the fitness measures would be the same. Based on these measures, women's peak heart rate made it difficult for many women to reach their exercise level intensity. A woman's maximum heart rate was consistently overestimated. Thankfully that belief has changed. There is now a "new" formula that provides a more accurate exercise peak heart rate for women.

I wrote this book to address the concerns specific to women as we age. You are never too old to exercise. That common phrase, "What you don't use, you lose!" carries a lot of weight regarding our bodies.

Our muscles help to move our bodies through space. As we age, we want our muscles to respond with ease and pain-free for as long as possible. Remember this is just the beginning in your quest to help jump-start your fitness journey. Truth be told, what is shared here, can be easily used for those who are younger and want to get started in their fitness pursuit. As a precaution, please consult with your physician when participating in any fitness program that puts your heart in a state of prolonged stress.

So, with that said, let's give this a go!

Two

MINDSET

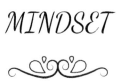

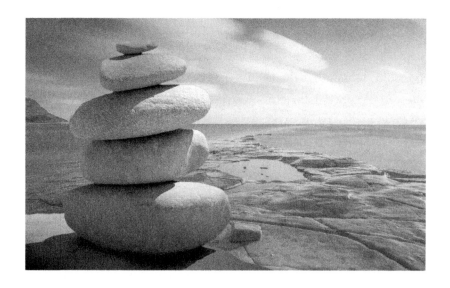

W hy explore a fitness mindset? Well, the mind is a strong muscle that can influence your performance towards the goals you set for yourself. Your fitness mindset is pivotal in the success or failure of your pursuit to reach your goal to become fit. First, framing your inner mind for fitness success is crucial to actually getting your body to respond positively to the work ahead.

When I think of mindset, I'm coaching my mind for success. I immediately think of the animated version of the 1970's Christmas show "Santa Claus is Coming to Town" where Claus sings the lyrics:

"You put one foot in front of the other and soon you'd be walking across the floor,

You put one foot in front of the other and soon you'd be walking out that door!"

I see these lyrics as a mantra and serve as motivation for me to generate action.

Moreover, if you want to succeed, you have to commit both mentally and physically to accomplish your goal. Keep in mind, that starting anything new has to start with that first step.

What is Your Reason for Fitness?

What mantra will serve as a positive motivation for you? Is it a family member, or a picture of what you see your future self be? Whatever it is, put it in a place where you can see this goal and be reminded of your "Why?" to become fit. See yourself charging onward to a life of fitness and propelling yourself forward towards success.

This will take mental work and commitment. Having a visual picture of yourself succeeding is a great way to stay motivated.

When you are faced with doubt or adversity in your fitness quest, acknowledge it, but do not let it side-track you before you even get started! Excuses will emerge… such as: "I don't have time! This is too hard! I don't have the right clothing, shoes, or equipment, to exercise!." I'm sure there are many more reasons which can be added to the list, but the cost of inaction is ultimately at the cost to your health. We are all human, invariably human nature is to place obstacles in our quest for success. So, do not let negative thoughts define your course of action. Individuals who pursue physical fitness as they grow older enjoy greater independence and are better able to maintain their quality of life.

Choosing this book is an indicator that you are interested in wanting to explore a life of fitness.

Explore the "What" and the "Why" in your reason for fitness? Your answer will be the key to your success. As you continue reading this book, give yourself that gentle reminder of the answer for your "What and/or why for wanting to improve your fitness level?"

What is fitness? There are numerous definitions in the fitness realm to answer this very question. However, I have included three fitness models to help define fitness. These models all have a common thread when defining fitness.

When I was in elementary school, fitness was broken down into:

- **Cardiovascular endurance** - the ability of the heart and lungs to work efficiently during timed aerobic exercise (stress test)
- **Flexibility**- where you were in a sitting position, legs straight out

in front of you while you reach towards your toes and beyond (if you could);

- **Muscular strength** - single, dynamic, explosive action muscles measured through the vertical jump, standing long jump, or grip test
- **Muscular endurance** - timed sit-ups and push-ups;
- **Balance and coordination** - the ability to hold a static balance on one leg and the ability to maintain your equilibrium while the body is in motion.
- **Body composition** - the measurement of the percentage of body fat taken in specific areas of the body.

The combination of these components helped to determine an individual's level of fitness. However remember, there is no one test that can truly measure how fit an individual is.

Campbell, N., De Jesus, S. & Prapavessis, H. (2013), defines fitness, as "Physical fitness is defined as one's ability to engage in daily activities with optimal performance, with the management of disease, fatigue, and stress and reduced sedentary behavior."

According to the National Institute on Aging, target elements of fitness as individuals age are:

- **Endurance** - participation in aerobic activities for at least 20 minutes to increase breathing and heart rate. This will help with maintaining your ability to execute activities of daily living and improve your ability to maintain sustained physical demands if needed.
- **Strength** - incorporating sustained resistance through the full range of motion

- **Balance (both static and dynamic balance)** - engaging the muscle groups to help us stay upright and controlled as we move our body through space
- **Flexibility** - keeping our muscles, joints, and ligaments supple and allowing the ability to go through the full range of motion with relative ease.

Fitness constitutes more than one element and requires full engagement in all these areas to be fully fit. Consistently engaging in all areas will improve your level of fitness, help maintain general independence and improve your quality of life.

RECIPE FOR FITNESS SUCCESS

To design a recipe for fitness success, you first need to establish a positive mindset towards wanting to live a fit and healthy lifestyle. You need to have a clear vision of what you will look like in the future as you accomplish your fitness goals. Be patient with yourself and have perseverance when setbacks occur. It is important to have fortitude and resilience with setbacks as you continue to pursue your fitness goals.

Remember this is a journey that will take time. Your consistency with:

- application towards your fitness program
- dedication to participate fully
- perseverance and resilience even when you encounter setbacks
- patience with your progress and keeping that positive attitude to keep you motivated is key to your fitness success!

Surround yourself with love, family, and friends who will support your journey to keep your mind and body as healthy as you can for as long as you can, to maintain and improve your quality of life. There is a level of physical stress the body needs to experience in order to build endurance and slowly build itself up to become a healthy and fit body.

The common threads used to define fitness are cardiovascular endurance, strength, balance, flexibility, and body composition. Consistent active engagement in all these components is fitness. Therefore these components aid in one's ability to:

- Confidently engage in activities of daily living freely
- Have confidence and ease to move through space without the fear of falling
- Maintain quality of life as pain-free as possible, therefore making life worth living and
- Continued general independence

as you grow older with grace and thrive with a joy for living.

Three

BODY IMPACT/BODY TRANSITIONS

How we think about aging paves our perception of the future. It's inevitable, that as we get older our bodies grow weaker and slow down. However, we should strive to keep our bodies as healthy as possible as we age, for as long as possible. Our life experiences helped to shape who we are in the present day. These experiences also impact how we view ourselves, and our bodies in the past, as well as the here and now.

Be mindful, that these past experiences do not define who you will be or strive to be in the near future!

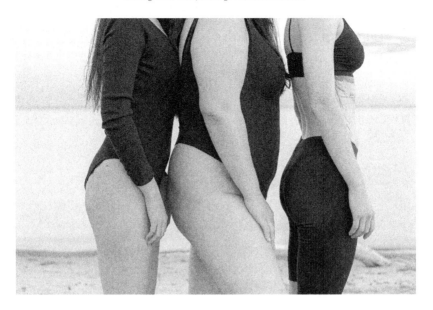

BODY TYPES

Let's consider our different body types as we age. The body's metabolism is different for each body type, therefore our body type should influence our choices in the type, quality, and quantity of fuels to consume when exercising. This practice of food choices will sway your pursuit of losing, gaining, or maintaining weight.

Do you remember the three different body types we learned during Health class in school?

Well, they are as follows:

- **Ectomorph** - is characterized as being naturally thin and having a fast metabolism. Their fast metabolism makes it difficult for this individual to gain weight.

- **Endomorph** - is characterized as an "apple-shaped" body. This individual usually has more stored fat, particularly around the stomach area, and can easily gain weight.
- **Mesomorph** - is characterized as the "hourglass figure", with broader shoulders, a slim waist, and larger hips. There is a tendency for greater muscle mass rather than excess fat tissue.

Itohan Esekheigbe presents another model, where there are greater differences in the female body types. These body types are divided into seven distinct categories. Esekheigbe, I. (August 12, 2021). "The 7 Most Common Female Body Types" are as follows:

- **Hourglass**-women with this body type have a narrow waist, their chests and hips are curvy and are the same or similar in size
- **Pear Shaped** - women with this body type have wider hips than their chest and shoulders
- **Rectangular** - women with this body type have their hips, waist, and bust with very similar measurements
- **Apple shape** - women with this body type have an undefined waist, and their busts are larger than the hips
- **Oval** - women with this body type have a full midsection with small breasts, their hips are narrow and their shoulders aren't broad.
- **Athletic** - women with this body type have a narrow waist, shoulder, and hips that are muscular and similar in size
- **Diamond** - women with this body type have broader hips with a fuller midsection. Their shoulders and bust are smaller than their hips.

Please take heart in knowing, that there is no "perfect body!" Defining a perfect body is what is perfect for you, regardless of what others think!

Considering the classification of body type, as we grow older "every-one's" metabolism slows down and we gain weight easier regardless of our body type. Our vision changes and our hearing isn't as acute as it once was. Walking up and down stairs takes a wee bit longer. Our hand grip isn't as strong to twist the lid off that pesky jelly jar with ease. Bending over to pick up something we dropped can elicit a groan as the pain receptors are triggered. Balancing can seem scary because of the fear of falling. Waking up in the morning takes a little longer. It takes time to get the blood flowing, get the joints lubricated, and allow the pain to subside. These are very valid concerns that can and will affect the quality of life. But it doesn't have to be that way. We have the ability to reverse or slow down the process of aging through conscious consistent participation toward a healthy and fit lifestyle.

SARCOPENIA

As we age we lose muscle mass which contributes to our diminishing strength. This loss of muscle mass and muscle quality as we age are known as sarcopenia. The European Working Group on Sarcopenia in Older People (EWGSOP, established in 2019) helped to develop the broad clinical definition of Sarcopenia which is currently used worldwide. Sarcopenia is a disease that progressively changes the body composition and directly affects the muscle quality and muscle mass of an individual when aging. This disease affects both men and women equally. The effects of sarcopenia can directly affect one's quality of life thereby impacting an individual's ability to perform activities of daily living. This can result in loss of independence and needing long-term care.

Symptoms of sarcopenia can be characterized as muscle weakness, loss of stamina, difficulty performing activities of daily living, poor balance, and falls. The sooner sarcopenia is identified, the better the opportunity is to address the muscle weakness and loss sooner. The longer poor muscle mass is ignored, the greater the probability the muscle status may lead to significant health impairments. Check with a physician or health care provider to determine if you or a loved one has sarcopenia.

One form of screening for sarcopenia is by assessing:

- Strength - grip strength
- Chair Stand - stand up and sit down as many times as you can
- Muscle Mass - measurement of appendicular lean muscle mass
- 400 meter/approximately 13 feet walk - walking on a treadmill and completing in 6 minutes or less

The body's peak level of performance occurs approximately around 15-30 years of age depending on activity levels. With aging, sarcopenia can affect people in their 30's and beyond. Muscles are designed to move the body through space. Consequently, with the loss of muscle quality and muscle mass, a decrease in the number and size of muscle fibers causes the muscle to thin, causing muscle atrophy and muscle weakness. Taking a closer look at muscles, it can be broken down into two types of fibers:

Slow-twitch muscle fibers - these muscle fibers are associated with resistance against fatigue and help to maintain strength output for longer periods of time. The slow-twitch muscle fibers are less affected by the aging process.

Fast-twitch muscle fibers - these muscle fibers are used for explosive movement and fatigue quicker than their counterpart Slow-twitch muscle fibers. The fast-twitch is greatly affected by the process of aging.

These muscle fibers help to determine the quality of movement. Note, after the age of 40 men's fitness levels decline at a faster rate than women's regardless of their physical activity level. Being physically inactive and eating an unhealthy diet, can result in obesity and allows the onset of sarcopenia.

Fortunately, the symptoms of sarcopenia can be reduced or reversed. The primary treatment for sarcopenia is resistance or strength training. This is crucial for women to know, that in order to slow down and reverse sarcopenia they should use some sort of resistance or strength training. Key practices to follow in treating sarcopenia:

- You must perform the proper number, intensity, and frequency of resistance/strength training to get the benefits necessary to decrease the symptoms of sarcopenia. Working with a Physical Therapist or trainer is key for an exercise plan.
- Participate in regular physical daily activity.
- Eat a healthy diet with high-quality proteins. The target range for protein consumption is approximately 20-35 grams of protein each meal.
- Get routine physicals. Check with your health care provider for the appropriate number of routine physicals in a year.

Remember, in order to decrease the effects of sarcopenia, regain muscle mass and improve muscle quality, the exercises executed need to engage the large muscle groups with active resistance, through the full range of motion. The intensity of the exercises needs to be completed within a specific time allotment in order to trigger the benefits of the efforts of the resistance.

BEYOND MENOPAUSE

Menopause is the natural part of aging for women. Natural menopause occurs in three stages.

- Perimenopause
- Menopause
- Postmenopause

Perimenopause for some women can occur in their thirties. However, the common age for perimenopause is usually in their forties. Perimenopause is typically a clinical diagnosis. In this stage, a woman's monthly menstruation is irregular and becomes dysregulated. The levels of estrogen increase. Common symptoms of perimenopause and menopause are:

- Hot flashes - Sudden flush of warmth around the face and upper body lasting between a couple of seconds, a few minutes, or longer. They can occur several times a day or several times a month.
- Night sweats - Occurrence of hot flashes during sleep.
- Cold flashes - Chills, cold feet, or shivering after the body starts to cool down from an episode of hot flashes.
- Vaginal changes - Urgent need to urinate, vaginal dryness, low libido, vaginal discomfort during sex due to vaginal dryness.

- Emotional changes - Mood swings, mild depression, irritability
- Difficulty sleeping - Usually due to hot flashes during sleep.

Perimenopause is sometimes confused with menopause because the symptoms are similar. The start of menopause occurs when monthly menstruation ceases. The hormonal control of the pituitary gland diminishes and the levels of estrogen and progesterone drop. This time is usually seen as the end of the reproductive years. The typical age for menopause is around the mid-forties or early fifties.

Post Menopause is marked after one year without menstrual bleeding. There are less frequent and powerful hot flashes. During post-menopause, there is a fluctuation of progesterone and lower levels of estrogen. This puts women at a greater risk of osteoporosis, sarcopenia, and heart disease.

In order to offset the detrimental effects of menopause, consistent exercise for approximately two hours per week; for 20-30 minutes per day. Health professionals in the field of fitness highly recommend specific consistent exercise to help with symptom relief, self-esteem boost, build bone density, weight management, and support muscle quality, and muscle size. Always check with your health care provider to determine if participating in activities that place the heart under consistent stress is appropriate.

BONE HEALTH

Our bones help to create the internal frame for our bodies and help maintain our shape while in motion. Bones are made up of livings cells and tissues which are in a constant state of change. This change allows the skeletal system to undergo a self-regeneration process called remodeling. Remodeling is a process that removes old bones and replaces them with new ones. At the age of approximately 50 years, we start losing bone faster than we can rebuild it.

As we look at our bones, we need to consider the importance of bone density. Bone density refers to the amount of minerals, specifically calcium and Phosphorus, within the bone. The measure of bone density serves as an indicator of the likelihood that the bone will fracture. Through the natural process of aging our bones slowly leech out these minerals causing the bone to become more porous. Consequently, this results in bone weakening. This bone deterioration lowers bone density, compromises the bone, and increases the probability of bone fracture. Furthermore, when women reach menopause the likelihood of bone loss density increases due to the loss of estrogen.

The importance of keeping our bones strong as we age cannot be understated! Half of all women and a quarter of men over the age of 50, raise the concern that they will become more prone to breaking their bones due to bone density loss. However, we do have steps that we can do to help preserve our bone health. Strategies to support bone health are:

- Consuming anti-inflammatory foods such as berries, fatty fish, avocado, tomatoes, turmeric, grapes, mushrooms, green tea, broccoli, peppers, tomatoes, lentils and kale, dark chocolate and cocoa

- Consulting with your physician for possible diet supplements
- Avoid over processes foods and excessive consumption of sugary sweets
- Keep alcohol consumption in moderation
- Get plenty of sleep
- Active and regular participation in **weight-bearing exercises** such as walking, running, **strength exercises** such as resistance bands, and weight lifting. Staying physically active and having an exercise plan that is tailored specifically for your needs is key to your fitness success.

Exercise plays a pivotal role in keeping our bones strong. Particularly strength training and weight-bearing exercises are key to keeping our bones healthy. The resistance exercises should include all muscle groups. All the resistance level needs to cause muscle fatigue after 12-15 repetitions in order to help increase muscle mass, muscle quality, and bone density. Free weights, weight machines, or the use of your own body weight are ways to use resistance.

The Physical Activity Key Guideline for Substantial Health Benefits for Adults/Older Adults created by the U.S. Department of Health and Human Services recommends:

- Muscle strengthening involves all major muscle groups at moderate or high intensity for 2 or more days a week.
- Balance exercise 3 times per week

A more comprehensive explanation regarding exercises will be discussed in the chapter called "Ready Set, Go!"

Four

DIET SMARTS

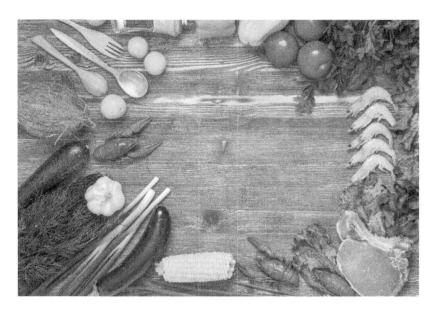

When I heard the word diet, I used to think it meant depriving oneself of eating meals to lose weight. Therefore

I used to say, "I don't believe in diets!"

However, with age comes wisdom. Working within the field of fitness I have found that I needed to gain further knowledge in this area. Diet exploration helped me gain a better perspective on the importance of what constitutes a healthy diet. Generally speaking, a diet is what we eat to fuel our bodies. It's the types, quality, and quantity of foods that we consume that determine whether it is beneficial or detrimental to our health.

Growing up in the 1960's we were taught the importance of USDA's "Food Guide Pyramid". Guidelines were given on the recommended types of foods that should be eaten in a day. As time marched forward, this model was found to be too simple and left too much ambiguity in the interpretation of the guidelines. In 2011 the Food Guide Pyramid was retired and replaced with MyPlate.

The MyPlate guidelines used the graphic of a plate divided into sections for the portions of vegetables, proteins, fruits, grains, and dairy. These portions would be similar to ½ produce, ¼ complex carbohydrates, and 1/4 proteins. Consumption in all food groups would ensure a balanced diet. These new dietary guidelines provided a more healthy and balanced diet.

For many individuals, struggling to reach that "ideal" weight can be very frustrating. "Dieters," thought the only way to reach their "ideal weight" is through "dieting". Bouncing from one diet plan to another in hopes the plan will live up to their claims, proved to be taxing to the body and in some cases could lead to death. Let me clarify by stating; "Some diets can be good to practice while other diets can be life-threatening!" Extreme caution should always be taken before choosing to participate in a weight loss program through dieting. Do your research on the diet program. Furthermore, talk with your physician/health care provider to ensure you will experience the most advantageous outcome in engaging in a diet plan to improve your quality of life and ensure your fitness level will not be compromised.

I have included the top 5 best diets for 2022 according to US News and World Report. Choices on the 5 best diets had to meet specific criteria to determine their rankings. The detailed ranking criteria can be found in the article from US News and World Report. Please note, that I do not necessarily endorse participation in any one of the diets described. I have included them strictly as examples of diets currently being practiced. They are as follows:

- **Mediterranean Diet** - emphasis on low consumption of red meat, sugar, and saturated fats. High value on fruits, vegetables, beans, legumes, nuts, whole grains, olive oil, fish, and seafood. There are no guidelines for portion size or caloric ranges.
- **DASH (Dietary Approaches to Stop Hypertension) Diet** - this plan is created so the individual can choose foods to help control high blood pressure (hypertension). Emphasis is on the consumption of foods rich in potassium, calcium, magnesium, fiber, and protein. Foods such as vegetables, fruits, whole grains, fish, poultry, low-fat dairy products, beans, and nuts. Servings are based on an individual's caloric needs.
- **Flexitarian Diet** - emphasis on consumption of plant-based products, fruits, vegetables, beans, lentils, whole grains, dairy, and seasonings. The meal plan includes five-week breakfast, lunch, dinner, and snack recipes using five main ingredients. Substitutions are allowed for easy-to-follow recipes and flexibility in meal plans. This plan allows for eating out. The daily total caloric intake for all

three meals with snacks is approximately 1,500.

- **MIND (Mediterranean-Intervention for Neurodegenerative Delay)** this diet is a combination of the Mediterranean and DASH that takes the best ideas from each plan to focus on foods specific to brain health. Emphasis on consumption of whole grains, attention to green leafy vegetables, fruits, nuts, fish, and poultry.
- **Mayo Clinic Diet** - consists of two phases: "Lose It!" where individuals learn the skill of counting calories in order to lose or maintain weight through healthy eating. During the first two weeks, eating out is discouraged, eating while watching television is not allowed, sugar is restricted except sugar from fruits, minimizing meat and full-fat dairy. Following the two-week period, the "Live It" phase begins. In this phase, instead of counting calories, portion size becomes the focus.

I personally think that adhering to the dietary guidelines for nutrition put forth by the USDA (United States Department of Agriculture) and the Department of Health and Human Services is a great way to plan a meal that is a balanced diet. When I cook, I try to use mostly organic foods, stay away from processed foods and minimize my sugar intake. I like to cook my own meals because I am aware of what and how the meal is created. The following is an example of my menu for a day:

Breakfast - a glass of water. I usually have a bowl of fruits (i.e., blueberries, bananas, strawberries, cherries, and/or white nectarine), and a cup of mixed nuts for a snack. Jasmine tea with vanilla almond milk. An alternative fruit bowl would be to make a fruit smoothie that would have blended fresh fruit, spinach, and vanilla almond milk.

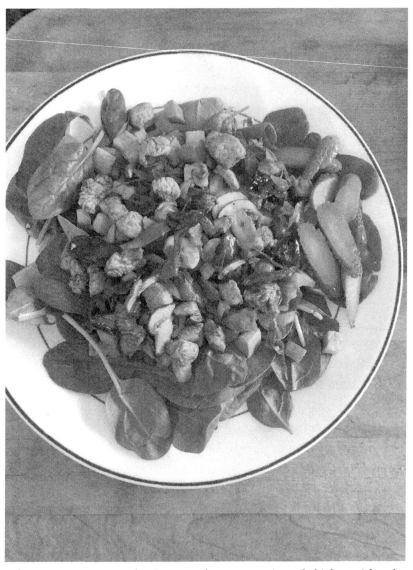

Sweet potatoes, sauteed onions, mushrooms, marinated chicken with red cabbage and onions, with a side of dill pickles

Lunch - Spinach Marinated Chicken Bowl
    200 grams cubed oven-roasted sweet potatoes

200 grams sauteed marinated chicken

150 grams of fresh spinach

100 grams of sliced sauteed mushrooms

25 grams of marinated red cabbage and red onions

5 sliced cherry tomatoes

3 sliced pickles

Water and jasmine tea with vanilla almond milk

Dinner -

100 grams sauteed lean ground turkey

250 grams fried (grapeseed oil) cubed potatoes

100 grams raw sliced carrots

Water and jasmine tea with almond milk

A healthy diet plays an important role in health and fitness, but diet alone is not enough to stay healthy. Daily consistent participation in exercise paired with diet helps to create a more effective healthy and fit lifestyle.

SUGARS

"Mmmm! I just love sugary sweets, pastries, cookies, baked goods, ice cream and more!" But as I embrace a more healthy lifestyle, I know I cannot let sugar run my life!

There are 4 common simple sugars:

- glucose - the most common sugar in plants
- fructose-sugar in fruit
- sucrose-table sugar,
- lactose-sugar in dairy.

Simple sugars are made of one sugar molecule.

Complex carbohydrates are formed from three or more sugar molecules and take longer to break down. The following are some examples of hidden sources of added sugar: Agave Nectar, Barley Malt Syrup, Brown Sugar, Brown Rice Syrup, Cane Juice, Cane Sugar, Coconut Sugar, Corn Syrup, Corn Syrup Solids, Evaporated Cane Juice, Evaporated Corn Sweetener, High Fructose Corn Syrup, Honey, Invert Sugar, Malt Syrup, Molasses, Palm Sugar, Raw Sugar, Rice Syrup, Turbinado Sugar, White Granulated Sugar. (Sassos, S., Oct. 29, 2020)

When sugar is consumed, Dopamine is triggered. Dopamine is a chemical released in the brain, a "feel good" neurotransmitter, that sends messages between nerve cells. Dopamine creates reinforcement to want more sugar in order to recreate the pleasure feeling experience.

Sugar consumption triggers hunger. Sugar is very addictive and at times difficult to curb or quit from craving. The more sugar we consume the more the body craves it. Food companies are aware of this fact and use this knowledge in the form of added sugars to their products. So stop and make a point to read the labels on processed foods to see if the amount of sugar it contains is worth feeding an addiction to sugar.

When we eat carbohydrates, our body converts them to glucose. This is the main source of fuel our body uses. Normally there are 4 grams (which is less than a teaspoon) of sugar coursing through our bloodstream. The body cannot keep more than 4 grams of sugar in the bloodstream. When there is an excess of sugar in the bloodstream our pancreas produces insulin. The insulin takes the excess sugar to the liver to be stored or taken to the muscles where it is converted into fat. When the body is constantly producing insulin due to excess sugar, the cells will become insulin resistant. This becomes a vicious cycle of insulin production which in turn triggers the release of more insulin. This is the cause of diabetes.

Consistent prolonged overindulgence in sugar consumption can lead to prediabetes, diabetes, obesity, risk of heart disease, skin, and cellular aging, fatty liver, heart disease, cognitive decline, and much more.

Sugar is naturally found in fruits and vegetables. Caution should be noted regarding foods with added sugars. This is adding sugar on top of existing sugar. Read the labels. Hidden sugars can be found in Breakfast cereals, yogurt, condiments, and sugary drinks like soda, sports drinks, fruit juices, shakes, etc. Be a wise and informed consumer when it comes to foods and drinks you choose to consume. This awareness will help you to be more active in your food selections. live a healthy lifestyle and support you in your fitness journey.

WATER

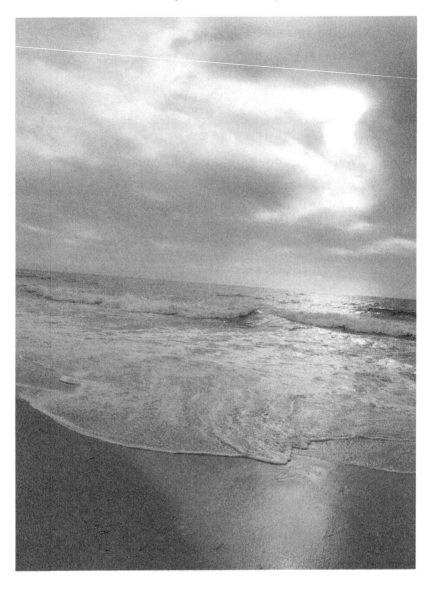

Our bodies are made up of 70% water. The benefits of water consumption cannot be overstated. Water helps to regulate the body's
temperature, cognitive abilities, and mood.

Thirst is the body's signal to quench the need for fluids. As we age our thirst signal declines. Consequently, seniors are at greater risk of dehydration. Therefore when thirst is recognized the body is already dehydrated. Simply put, dehydration occurs when you are consuming less water than your body needs.

A quick way to check if you're dehydrated is to do a "skin pinch" test on the top of your hand, palm side down. If the skin does not quickly rebound then this can serve as an indicator of dehydration. Another technique is checking the color of your urine. If the urine is pale or clear in color is a good indicator of being well hydrated. If it is dark colored with amber or brown tones you may be dehydrated.

Dehydration is dangerous no matter the individual's age. Symptoms of dehydration are muscle weakness, lethargy, dry mouth, headaches or dizziness, and low blood pressure. In severe instances of dehydration, symptoms can progress to fever, confusion, disorientation, increased urination, excessive sweating, and inability to keep fluids down. In these cases, the body is in crisis mode and immediate medical attention should be sought! Delays in this matter could lead to urinary and kidney problems, seizures, heat exhaustion or heat stroke, or death.

One way to keep hydrated is to set a timer to remind and train yourself to rehydrate. Always keep a bottle of water with you. Water can be enhanced with a slice of lemon or lime, infused with cucumber or fruit. The amount of water to consume varies with each individual. According to the National Council on Aging, "A good rule of thumb, take a ⅓ of your body weight and consume that number in fluid ounces. For example, if you weigh 150 pounds then you should drink 50 fluid ounces per day."

When we first wake up in the morning, drink water on an empty stomach. You could mix ¼ teaspoon of Himalayan salt or Celtic salt (or any salt rich in minerals) with 1 liter of water to replace the electrolytes lost during sleep. The electrolytes are lost through sweat and urination. Electrolytes are minerals that help with the pH balance within the body and support nerve signaling, muscle contraction, muscle cramping, and rehydration. You do not need to drink the whole liter all at once. It can be consumed throughout the day. If you have a history of hypertension, thyroid issues, or heart-related issues, always check with your physician to decide if drinking water with any salt is contraindicated.

Consumption of alcoholic drinks should be monitored and done in moderation. Alcoholic drinks serve more as a diuretic and increase dehydration.

Additionally, it is essential to remember your body needs more water when engaging in physical activity. Make sure to have your bottled water ready as you move from one exercise to another and take the time to rehydrate. You will find that you will have greater endurance and be in a better mood to complete your activity.

OBESITY

An individual is considered obese when their body mass index (BMI) is 30 or greater. BMI can be measured through skinfold caliper measurements, underwater weighing, or dual-energy x-ray imaging which are a little more affordable. BMI is strongly correlated to body fatness. When an individual's weight is greater than the recommended healthy allowance for the individual's height they are considered to be obese.

Studies have shown that obesity in the United States has grown significantly over the past twenty years. The data from the National Health and Nutrition Examination Survey revealed more than ⅓ of the population in our country is obese. People 60 years and older are more likely to be obese than young adults. Children between 2 through 19 years of age are considered clinically obese. A man's weight after 50 years of age tends to remain the same and decreases slightly between 60-74 years of age. Women tend to increase in weight until age 60 and gradually decrease weight thereafter.

Obesity occurs when more calories are consumed than the body burns off over a period of time. When an excess amount of calories frequently occurs, weight gain happens. The lack of physical activity contributes to obesity and other health-related problems.

Obesity means there is more visceral fat around vital organs. Visceral fat is where most toxins are stored. When visceral fat is converted into energy these toxins are released around the organs. Serious health problems can occur from obesity such as hypertension, diabetes, breathing issues, sleep pattern disruptions, and cancer.

The combination of diet and consistent daily participation in a fitness regimen aids an individual to lose weight and generate muscle mass necessary to decrease fat storage. Seek partnership with your medical health care provider to determine a healthy course of action to lose weight, monitor weight loss, and keep the weight off.

MEDICATIONS

As you get older your blood pressure may become high resulting in hypertension. Or maybe you have been diagnosed with diabetes, cancer, osteoporosis, etc. These are just a few physical health ailments that may potentially require medication to help your body stay within the normal range to stay "healthy".

If you are an individual who is taking medications, be aware of their side effects. The medication side effects (depending on the purpose of the medication) can negatively impact the efficiency of your heart and lungs before, during, or after exercise. Additionally, the medication could affect the proper outcome of your Target Heart Rate (THR) measures. The THR is the number we use to determine if you are working within the appropriate intensity zone to derive and improve your fitness. Working at your right intensity ensures your opportunity to meet your fitness goals will be completed in a safe manner.

Please note, be proactive to know as much as you can about the medications you are on, their functions, and how they impact your health. Your knowledge regarding your health is necessary to preserve your physical well-being. Speak with your physician or health care provider. Inform them that you will be participating in a fitness program and have created goals to improve your health and fitness.

Learn if there are any adverse side effects from the medication that could occur when you are participating in a fitness program/activity. These side effects could be life-threatening. Speaking with your physician or health care provider could help to address potential issues that may arise when you are exercising. Furthermore, you should know how to avoid these side effects as you engage in your pursuit of a healthier and fit lifestyle

Five

SLEEP

Q uality sleep is vital to living a fit and healthy life. Sleep allows the body to heal after a long, hard day of work. The heart and lungs are able to rest, blood pressure decreases and cardiac health improves, blood sugar is better regulated, and the growth hormone that aids in the growth and repair of muscles is more effective during sleep. After a good night's sleep, the body is energized, mental functioning improves, stress decreases in order to be able to handle the challenges of the day, and helps to reduce chronic inflammation.

The impact of inadequate sleep is as follows:

- Impairs memory and mental functioning
- Negatively impacts mood regulation
- Increases risk of heart disease
- Increase risk of high blood pressure
- Decreases the body's immune system to fight off infections

- Fatigue
- Weight gain
- Increased risk of injury
- Depression

According to the Centers for Disease Control and Prevention, the recommended average amount of sleep for adults and older adults is between 7-9 hours.

STRATEGIES FOR QUALITY SLEEP

Getting quality sleep can be a challenge. These are a number of healthy practices to train your body for sleep:

- **Design a consistent regular sleep schedule.** This means going to bed and waking up at the same time every day including weekends. This will train the body's inner circadian rhythm/cycle to regulate the sleep-wake cycle approximately every 24 hours.
- **Quality sleep environment.** Adjust the darkness of the room, the temperature of the room that will allow falling asleep easier, the types of pillows, sheets, and blankets needed for sleep, and the quiet environment.
- **Restrict eating at least 3 hours before scheduled bedtime.** Decreases discomfort of digestion before bedtime.
- **Avoid the use of technology at least 1 hour before bedtime.** This includes phones, computers, and televisions. The emission of blue light from these devices tricks the body by giving the impression that it is still daylight hours.

- **Avoid consumption of caffeine, alcohol, and nicotine before bedtime.** Caffeine is a stimulant, Alcohol creates lighter, lower quality sleep, and nicotine is a habit associated with daytime activities.
- **Exercise during the day, no later than 3 hours before bedtime.** This will allow adequate time for the body to relax before bedtime.

Six

FITNESS, IS ONLY A STEP AWAY

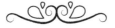

Before starting a fitness program check with your Physician/Health Care Professional to determine the appropriateness to engage in physical activities that will place stress on your heart and lungs for a prolonged aerobic stress state (i.e, 10 minutes or greater). You should exercise within your abilities and medical condition.

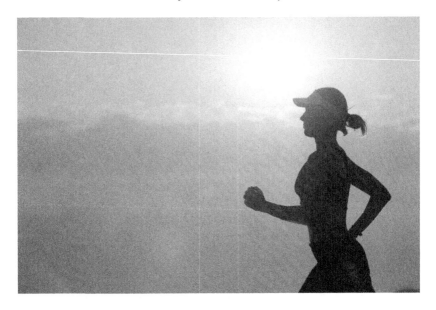

PHYSICAL ACTIVITY GUIDELINES FOR ADULTS/OLDER ADULTS

US Department of Health and Human Services: Physical Activity Key Guideline for substantial health benefits for adults/older adults:

- 150 minutes (2 ½ hours) per week of moderate-intensity activity or
- 75 minutes of high-intensity aerobic activity per week. Aerobic activity can be divided into a minimum of 10 minutes each spread throughout the week.
- Muscle strengthening involves all major muscle groups at moderate or high intensity for 2 or more days a week.
- Balance exercise 3 times per week
- Gradually increase to 300 minutes per week of moderate-intensity activity

ESTABLISHING FITNESS BASELINES

Knowing your fitness starting point or baseline is crucial to determine fitness growth during your fitness journey. Determining your target heart rate for peak performance would be a good place to begin. Listen to your body to give you an indication that you aren't overdoing your workouts.

There are four commonly used formulas used to determine Target Heart Rate (THR):

- **Fox Formula** (standard formula, used for both men and women):

220 - age = Maximum Heart Rate

- **Gulati Formula** (women only):

39

206 - (0.88 x age) = Maximum Heart Rate

- **HUNT Formula** (used for active men and women)

211 - (0.64 x age) = Maximum Heart Rate

- **Tanaka Formula** (used for men and women over 40 years of age)

208 - (0.7 x age) = Maximum Heart Rate

For the purposes of this book, I will be focusing on the Fox Formula and Gulati Formula.

Target Heart Rate is the measurement of exercise intensity on the cardiovascular system and is a range instead of a single number. The percentage calculations serve as a way to measure the type of exercise intensity.

The **Fox Formula** (the standard formula) is commonly used to determine Maximum Heart Rate. It was created in the late 1930's and is based on studies done on men when exercising.

The **Fox Formula** is as follows:
    Please note, that calculations for the Fox Formula are for a 50-year-old person.

220 (beats per minute) - age = Maximum Heart Rate (MHR)
    220 - 50 = 170 MHR

Maximum Heart Rate is the fastest the heart beats in a minute. Target Heart Rate (THR) is a range of numbers expressed in percentages used to determine how fast the heart is beating during exercise. The range we will be using is 60% - 85%. MHR is taken from the formula above.

MHR x percentage = Target Heart Rate (THR)
    170 x 0.6 = 102
    170 x. 0.85 = 144.5 rounding up to 145

When exercising, using the range of 60% - 85% of max heart rate, Target Heart Rate should be between 102-145 beats per minute.

This formula has been commonly used for decades. It has come under scrutiny because the foundation of the formula is based on an estimate from observation of raw and mean data collected on the men in the study.

Furthermore, this formula was used universally for men and women. It did not differentiate the differences between men and women. Women were thought of as being smaller men. Consequently, the Fox Formula used for women overestimated their target heart rate so women typically could not reach it.

We know the physiology of women is different than that of men. Martha Gulati, MD conducted a study that included 5,437 women 35 years and older to determine how their hearts responded to the treadmill exercise. The subjects were exercising for as long and hard as they could. Through this 20-year study, a more accurate gender-specific formula was created. Calculating the target heart rate for women has changed to get the most effective workout.

Gulati's formula is as follows:
    Using Gulati's Formula, the following calculations are done for a

50-year-old woman.
    206 minus(0.88 x age) = Maximum Heart Rate (MHR)
    206 - (0.88 x 50) = MHR
    206 - 44 = 162 MHR

Target Heart Rate (THR) is a range of numbers expressed in percentages used to determine how fast the heart is beating during exercise. The range we will be using is 60% - 85%. MHR is taken from the formula above.

MHR x percentage = Target Heart Rate (THR)
    162 x 0.6 = 97.2 rounding down 97 THR
    162 x 0.85 = 137.7 rounding up to 138 THR

When exercising, using the range of 60% - 85% of max heart rate, Target Heart Rate should be between 97-138 beats per minute.

Comparing the two formulas side-by-side:
        Fox's Formula vs Gulati's Formula-gender specific
    THR 102-145 bpm 97-138 bpm
        Reveals a difference of 5-7 beats per minute

Women this difference may not seem like a lot, but it is significant when you are attempting to reach your target heart rate particularly when you are working at 85% of your maximum heart rate. Remember that the target heart rate is calculated for sustained exercise activity, which is typically exercising at a minimum of 10-12 minutes.

I highly recommend using Gulati's formula when calculating your Target Heart Rate because it is gender specific. Also if you haven't been exercising regularly, focus on a goal of 60% of your THR. The

Center for Disease Control and Prevention recommends, "Move more and Sit Less!"

Furthermore, if you haven't been exercising at all, "Go low and start Slow!" per the recommendation of the US Department of Health and Human Services. If you have had a sedentary lifestyle and have not engaged in consistent regular exercise, you need to build up your endurance to protect your body from harm or injuries.

Listed are two alternative methods for taking your THR:

- **"Talk Test"** is a subjective measure of gauging how you are feeling while exercising. This test involves being able to engage in a conversation during a brisk exercise and breathing without gasping or laboriously taking a breath is an indicator of THR.
- **VO2 max or Aerobic Capacity** is usually done with a trained individual. This is a test that is done on a treadmill or stationary bike. Progressive resistance is used to determine the maximum capacity of oxygen consumed during an exercise interval. Termination of the assessment occurs to voluntary exhaustion.
- **Borg's Rate of Perceived Exertion (RPE)** is another subjective measure that can be self-administered or assessor administered. The subject is asked how they feel as they are working out to gauge their level of exertion. The scale ranges from 6 (being the easiest) - 20 (maximal exertion)

These aforementioned tests of gauging your Target Heart Rate are not an exhaustive list, however, it is a good place to start.

FITNESS ACCOUNTABILITY QUESTIONNAIRE

This questionnaire is designed to trigger your "what" and your "why" for pursuing a healthy fitness lifestyle. Additionally, I hope it helps you to clarify your focus on your fitness journey and be able to create realistic, attainable fitness goals for yourself as you age. It would be a good idea to make a copy of the questionnaire or rewrite the questions with your answers so can refer to them periodically as reminders of your fitness pursuits.

Your answers to the following questions are for your eyes only. Please take the time to answer each question as honestly as possible. If you choose, you have the option to share the questionnaire with others who can help you stay accountable and motivate you to fulfill your fitness goals. Additionally, you can always refer back to the answers to these questions to remind you of your goals for a more fit and healthier lifestyle.

- **Are you currently engaging in any type of physical activity related to health and fitness? If so, what are they? How many times in a day, week, or month are you actively participating in the activity?**

- _____

- **What is your reasoning for becoming fit? Is it to look and feel good? Is it to lose weight? Is it so you can have the strength and stamina to keep up with your** grandkids? Maybe have the strength and endurance to go up and down stairs without being winded? Is it to maintain your quality of life and level of independence?

- What is your baseline or beginning level of fitness? The purpose of knowing your baseline fitness level is to give you a starting point for your fitness journey. It will also show how much growth you experienced in a given period of time.

  - ---

- How do you see yourself a month from now? In Six months? In a year?

  - ---

- Is your goal attainable? Is it realistic? If not, why not?

  - ---

Seven

EQUIPMENT ESSENTIALS

GUIDE TO DRESSING FOR FITNESS

T his section is a simple guideline for choosing appropriate equipment as you start your fitness journey. Please be aware, that I am not endorsing any brand of fitness equipment or fitness attire. I am merely giving general guidelines to use when preparing for your fitness quest.

Whether you are walking, running, hiking, or playing on a court, wearing the appropriate kind of shoes for the activity is important to protect your feet. Your shoes are your key to comfort, they will help to decrease foot fatigue, help with body alignment, and support you during activity.

For many weight-bearing types of exercise, the appropriate choice of shoes is paramount to your feet's health. There are many different types of athletic shoes out there. Shoes are designed for specific activities such as basketball, baseball, dance, running, weight training, tennis, etc. Be aware, that not all shoes are created equal, nor do they serve the same support when moving from one activity to another. So choosing the correct shoes for any given activity does affect athletic performance outcomes.

Your feet are unique to you and the selection of a shoe should reflect where your foot needs support, ie., arch supports of fallen arches, heel strike cushions to support heels from the repetitive pounding of heels when running, pronation, or rolling of the foot. When you are looking for the appropriate athletic shoe, speak with a knowledgeable sales associate. They will be able to guide you to the right place to look and answer questions that you may have regarding the quality of the pair. When trying on shoes, make sure to wear the same type of socks you will be using when you are exercising. The shoe should have a comfortable fit as soon as you put them on and when you walk around the store. They should <u>not</u> have to be "broken in" before they start to feel comfortable. Your feet are the foundation of your body, do not skimp on the quality of your shoes.

Regardless of what type of fitness activity you choose, your clothing should not restrict your range of motion. Moisture-wicking materials help to pull the sweat from the body, dry quicker and help to keep the body cool. If you are outdoors, hiking, walking, or running, there is clothing designed to protect the skin from sun damage. Hats and sunglasses are also a must to protect the skin and eyes from damage from ultraviolet light. Choose the clothing appropriate for the season and weather variability.

Include sunscreen for outside activities. Sunscreen with SPF (Sun Protection Factor) of at least 30 is recommended. The SPF number gives the effective time (in minutes) of protection from ultraviolet rays. Try to reapply sunscreen before the time runs out. The higher the SPF the longer the protection.

Fitness trackers, depending on the device, have the ability to document the number of steps taken, keep track of heart rate, and distance of exercise, document the amount of time exerted during exercise and can differentiate between walking, running, cycling, and much more. They can come in the form of a watch, or chest strap, or even your cell phone can act as a fitness tracker.

HOME GYM vs GYM MEMBERSHIP

Included are some things to ponder if you are considering whether to invest in a home gym or pay for a monthly gym membership.

HOME		vs	GYM
PRO	**CON**	**PRO**	**CON**
Convenient, no Travel time or parking to worry about	Storage of equipment	Variety of equipment Machines & Free Weights available	Wait time to use Equipment if in use from another patron
Done in privacy of your home	Limited variety of equipment	Dedicated space	Need to be trained to operate machines appropriately
No wait time for use of equipment	No trainer, no spotter	Trainers for guidance and form correction available	Cost of monthly gym membership
Time flexibility. You own the equipment.	Initial cost of purchasing equipment.	People to help with spotting.	Closures for holidays
Can have a variety of fitness classes on-line, participation in the privacy of your own home.	Cost prohibitive. No trainer/teacher available to pose questions for clarifications.	Variety of fitness classes available in the gym. You can speak with instructor if you have questions	There may be an added cost to participate in the classes. Time offerings may be inconvenient.

Please note, this chart is only a short list of pros and cons for both gym considerations and can be easily added onto. Ultimately whatever mode of gym you choose, make sure the gym benefits outweigh the negatives towards your fitness journey.

Be strategic and informed, your fitness journey does not have to be long, boring, or tedious. That would be a recipe for disaster! Choose an activity that you find interesting and will keep you motivated to do even when no one is watching.

If you are interested to be a part of a fitness group and want to have a bit more accountability here are a few suggestions:

- Explore live online workouts, fitness classes, yoga, etc.
- Invest in a fitness coach
- Check your hospital for fitness offerings.
- Check your local recreation center for fitness programs, your local church, etc.

Whatever fitness form you choose to engage in, remember you do have to challenge yourself in order to reap the benefits of fitness!

Eight

READY, SET, GO!

WARM-UPS

L et's get your blood pumping to your muscles, lubricate your joints for the full range of motion and prepare your body and mind for movement. Your warm-up should start from head to toe or vice versa. It really doesn't matter which direction you start with, just remember which reference point you started with and continue until you have stretched and warmed up all your major muscle groups. Your stretches should always include all major muscle groups. The warm-ups should last between 8 to 10 minutes. A great way to warm up is to music. Start slow and steady and avoid bouncing when you stretch your muscles.

To stretch your muscle groups, a good rule of thumb to follow:

- Breath normally throughout your stretching as you go through your full range of motion
- A stretch should be held for a minimum of five seconds
- A stretch should be mildly uncomfortable and should not cause pain when held

LET'S GET OUR BODIES MOVING!

As a beginner, you really don't need any special equipment to start. But, I highly recommend investing in a good pair of fitness shoes that will support you throughout your workout.

Just starting out? Resist the temptation to "Go All Out"! Your mind may want to start full out, and "get-fit-quick", but your body is not conditioned for the exercise demands! Remember your current ongoing lifestyle of inactivity contributes to your level of minimal fitness. It will take time to start or regain your level of healthy fitness.

Keep in mind, you will need to build your positive mindset as previously discussed in the Mindset section. Framing your inner mind for fitness success is crucial to prepare your body to respond positively to the work ahead. As your ability to engage in exercise increases, your confidence in your body's ability will also increase.

Your body needs to be trained for endurance. Fortunately, your body does quickly respond to the demands given. Remember to start out slow! Choose an activity you enjoy that will motivate you to keep your body moving. Is it dancing? Can you dance through one song or two without feeling "wiped out"? Is it walking? Can you walk around your house once without getting winded? How about your yard? Your block? What is your favorite activity and can you apply this concept? Is it hiking, cycling, or swimming?

Variety is the spice of life, so vary your activities to keep it fresh, and interesting and you know will keep you engaged. For example, consider swapping walking one day with dancing to your favorite music the next day. Or swim and switch it up with water aerobics.

Once you have been able to successfully engage in your activity of choice for at least 5 minutes each day, then increase your activity to 10 minutes/ day. Have a target to build your endurance for at least 20 minutes/day. In order to increase your activity intensity, you have to challenge yourself.

Have a realistic plan, and challenge yourself to see if you can "do at least one more." For example, if it's balancing on one leg, can you balance on one leg for one more second or complete one more set? Or maybe pushing a resistance band through your full range of motion one more time without compromising your form?

As a reminder, The US Department of Health and Human Services created the "Physical Activity Key Guideline for Substantial Health Benefits for Adults/Older Adults". The recommendations are as follows:

- 150 minutes (2 ½ hours) per week of moderate-intensity activity or
- 75 minutes of high-intensity aerobic activity per week. Aerobic activity can be divided into a minimum of 10 minutes each spread throughout the week.
- Muscle strengthening involves all major muscle groups at moderate

or high intensity for 2 or more days a week.
- Balance exercise 3 times per week
- Gradually increase to 300 minutes per week of moderate-intensity activity

DAILY LIVING EXERCISES

- **Chair Sit:**
- Choose a chair (dining room chair) that is firm. Option to have armrests.
- Standing in front of your chair and facing away.
- Stand up with control and sit down with control.
- Do at least 5 stand up - sit down sets in a row without stopping. If you have a chair with armrests, you can use it to keep your balance as you complete the sets. If not you can hold onto the side base of your chair to help keep your balance as you complete the sets.
- Do not hold your breath, you should be able to maintain your normal breathing cadence.
- This exercise works:
- Core (abdominal) muscle group
- Upper body
- Legs
- Back
- Balance
- flexibility
- **Chair Sit Variation**: Stand up, Sit down, Reach
- Same procedure as above, however, there is the added motion of reaching.

Both arms reach out in front of you at shoulder height. Reach out to the sides of your body; reach high above your head; reach down to your toes.

- **Getting up and down from the floor:**
- Sitting on the floor, rug or mat proceed to stand up.
- Sit back down with smoothness and control. If you need support, position yourself close to the wall, or have a sturdy piece of furniture you can use to hold on to as you raise and lower yourself.
- This exercise works:
- Core (abdominal) muscle group
- Upper body
- Legs
- Back
- Balance
- Full body strength
- Trunk and hip flexibility

- **Wall push-up:**
- Facing the wall straight arms, palms flat on the wall shoulder height
- Standing with legs hips width apart
- Body straight and tight through the full range of motion
- Bend at the elbows and try to touch your nose to the wall
- Return to starting position
- This exercise works:
- Upper body strength
- Shoulder, elbow, and wrist flexibility
- Core (abdominal) muscle group
- Ankle flexibility

- **Walking up and down stairs:**
- Standing upright, take your normal stride to ascend
- Handrails can be used for balance if needed
- This exercise works:
- Upper and lower body strength
- Strengthens glute muscles
- Cardiovascular fitness
- Balance
- coordination

BALANCE EXERCISES

- **Standing on one foot**
- Use only as needed. Using the back of a chair or furniture that you can lightly hold onto to aid with balance. Build endurance to stand on one foot without holding on to any furniture.
- Tighten your abdominals, legs, and glutes
- Repeat with the other foot
- **Raising and lowering on tiptoes**
- Standing with hips-width apart feet flat on the ground
- Raise up to your tip toes and try to hold for a count of three
- Lower back down to flat feet
- Repeat

- **Standing with legs apart; upper body sway**
- swaying upper body, changing weight from one leg to the other

- **Walking heel-to-toe**

- **Yoga or Tai Chi classes**

Balance exercises should be done 3 times per week.

RESISTANCE EXERCISES

Resistance exercises are to help build muscle quality and muscle mass. The specific number, intensity, and frequency of the resistance exercise are key to experiencing fitness benefits. The resistance exercises should include all muscle groups. All the resistance level needs to cause muscle fatigue after 12-15 repetitions in order to help increase muscle mass, muscle quality, and bone density. Free weights, weight machines, or the use of your own body weight are ways to use resistance.

Muscle strengthening involves all major muscle groups at moderate or high intensity for 2 or more days a week.

AEROBIC EXERCISES

Aerobic exercise is the increase of heart and lung functions through physical activity. Participation in aerobic exercises should last between 10-30 minutes in duration to gain fitness benefits. A great way to get your aerobic exercise is after each meal to do a brisk walk for a minimum of 10 minutes each.

- 150 minutes (2 ½ hours) per week of moderate-intensity activity or
- 75 minutes of high-intensity aerobic activity per week. Aerobic activity can be divided into a minimum of 10 minutes each spread throughout the week.
- Gradually increase to 300 minutes per week of moderate-intensity activity

Aerobic activities should be within moderate to intense levels to improve cardiovascular fitness. Types of aerobic activities would be brisk walking, running, dancing, swimming, water aerobics, hiking, interval weight training, cycling, etc. The ideal step range is between 7,000-9,000 steps per day. At least 3,000 steps need to be aerobic to be optimal. Walking is one of the best ways to increase your heart rate.

COOL DOWN

Your cool down is also very important to protect your muscles from injury after your active participation in exercising. It will give your mind the opportunity to find balance after intense focus on your exercise performance. Take the time to adequately stretch all your large muscle groups. Drink plenty of water to replace what you have lost through sweating, urination, and digestion. Your cool down should take no less than 10 minutes to complete.

SAMPLE FITNESS SCHEDULE FOR THE WEEK

This is an example of a fitness schedule that you can use to kick-start your fitness journey. There are numerous ways in which this schedule can be modified to meet your fitness goals.

Walking is one of the best ways to start your moderate-intensity or high-intensity activity. An easy way to determine if you are hitting your target heart rate is to use I like to use a combination of the:

- **"Talk Test"** - is a subjective test where you are gauging how you feel while you are exercising. You should be able to carry on a conversation during a brisk walk, run, or cycling without gasping or having difficulty taking a breath.
- **Rate of Perceived Exertion** - is another subjective test, where you are gauging how you feel while you are exercising. This was originally Borg's Rate of Perceived Exertion which had a scale ranging from 6 (easiest) to 20 (hardest). I modified the scale that ranges from 1 to 10. A score of 1 is extremely easy and 10 is extremely difficult. You would want to aim for a score between 7-9 for your target heart rate.

This sample schedule includes:

- resistance/strength exercises 2 times per week
- balance exercises 3 times per week
- moderate intensity aerobics every day. This is typically done after a meal to help with digestion and gives you the opportunity to go out in your neighborhood, walk the dog to enjoy the outdoors, or have a moment to get a breath of fresh air.

MON.	TUES.	WED.	THURS.	FRI.	SAT.	SUN.
	Resistance exercise 10-15 Minutes		Resistance exercise 10-15 Minutes			
Balance 5 minutes		Balance 5 minutes		Balance 5 minutes		
Lunch Walk 10 minutes	Lunch Walk 10 minutes	Lunch Walk 10 minutes	Lunch Walk 10 minutes	Lunch Walk 10 minutes	Lunch Walk 10 minutes	Lunch Walk 10 minutes
After Dinner Walk 15 minutes	After Dinner Walk 15 minutes	After Dinner Walk 15 minutes	After Dinner Walk 15 minutes	After Dinner Walk 15 minutes	After Dinner Walk 15 minutes	After Dinner Walk 15 minutes

I designed this sample fitness schedule to adhere to the recommendations put forth by the US Department of Health and Human Services: Physical Activity Key Guideline for substantial health benefits for adults/older adults. This is just a sample to help you in your design if you wish to create your own fitness schedule.

Nine

MUSCLE SORENESS

Muscle soreness can occur during and/or after each exercise which can impact your ability to workout. It is normal to experience natural muscle soreness when you first engage in a fitness program. Strategies to help offset muscle soreness is important to be able to participate fully towards your fitness goals.

There are two types of muscle soreness:

- acute muscle soreness - occurs during or immediately after exercise. This type of muscle soreness is easily resolved.
- Delayed Onset Muscle Soreness (DOMS) - occurs between 24-48 hours after an activity. This type of muscle soreness is due to microscopic tears in the muscle fibers and connective tissue during exercise.

A key to remember in muscle soreness is to keep moving. Start out with gentle dynamic movements such as big arm swings, and easy walking. The more exercise you do, the less soreness you will feel due to the muscle "rebound effect." This allows the muscle to adapt to stress, protect itself and get stronger!

STRATEGIES TO HELP WITH MUSCLE SORENESS

Some natural strategies to help ease muscle soreness:

- Drink plenty of water to help flush the toxins out of your muscles and keep your body hydrated. Keeping your body hydrated helps to reduce cramping and decreases inflammation.
- Warm Epsom salt bath - helps with relaxing the muscles. Soak for at least 12-20 minutes
- Foam roller - use on muscles that are sore. Foam rolling helps increase blood circulation within the area, increases muscle flexibility, or loosens tight achy muscles.
- Get a massage
- Drinking tart cherry juice, watermelon juice, pomegranate juice, and beet juice provides anti-inflammatory benefits. Foods such as eggs and dairy aid with muscle recovery, muscle repair, and muscle growth.
- After a workout, make sure to take the time to do gentle cool-down static stretches. A static stretch is held for at least 5 to 10 seconds.

When you engage in an exercise program, you will encounter soreness. However, your muscle soreness should not prevent you from doing your "normal activities of daily living." If this happens, you are overdoing it, you will need to ease up on your intensity but still participate in your exercising.

Remember you should be able to hit your target heart rate without compromising your ability to go about your day and function normally.

Ten

CONCLUSION

Awesome! A big heartfelt congratulations! You were able to successfully navigate through this fitness guidebook and gain some idea of where to begin.

Now is the time to execute your fitness journey through physical action. My hope is that you have been able to find useful information to guide you in your quest for fitness. Furthermore, my desire is to give you the fitness sense guidance as a beginner and provide you with the tools needed to start your fitness journey.

I would like to finish with two quotes:

"Motivation is what gets you started, habit is what keeps you going." Jim Ryun

"Dreams can come true if we have the courage to pursue them." Walt Disney

Remember you are investing in your future and contributing to

your overall health and well-being!

If you have found this book helpful please write a favorable review on Amazon.

Eleven

RESOURCES

MINDSET

B *alance Training.* (n.d.). Retrieved September 16, 2022, from https://www.topendsports.com/fitness/balance-training.htm

Campbell, N., Jesus, D. S., & Prapavessis, H. (2013). *Physical Fitness.* SpringerLink. Retrieved September 16, 2022, from https://link.springer.com/referenceworkentry/10.1007/978-1-4419-1005-9_1167?error=cookies_not_supported&code=d8f996b4-430b-45ba-a9d8-c35d94f53d60

Four Types of Exercise Can Improve Your Health and Physical Ability. (n.d.). *National Institute on Aging.* Retrieved September 16, 2022, from https://www.nia.nih.gov/health/four-types-exercise-can-improve-your-health-and-physical-ability

Santa Claus Is Comin' To Town. (1970). [Video]. DVD.

- YouTube. (n.d.). Retrieved September 16, 2022, from https://www.youtube.com/watch?v=nKUsZqBNzk

BODY IMPACT/ BODY TRANSITIONS

Hasan, M. (2022, July 28). *What are the 3 Female Body Types?* WOMS. Retrieved September 16, 2022, from https://worldofmedicalsaviours.com/female-body-types/

Female Body Types: *7 Of the Most Common Ones.* Retrieved September 16, 2022, from www.zikoko.com/her/7-different-female-body-shapes/

SARCOPENIA

Dunkin, M. (2020, July 19). *Sarcopenia With Aging.* Retrieved September 16, 2022, from www.webmd.com.

Thorpe, M. (2017, May 25). *How to Fight Sarcopenia: muscle loss due to aging.* www.healthline.com. Retrieved September 16, 2022, from https://www.healthline.com

Warner, J. (2005, July 25). *Fitness Level Declines Dramatically with Age: Exercise May Counteract Age-Related Decline in Physical Fitness.* www.webmd.com. Retrieved September 16, 2022, from https://www.webmd.com/fitness-exercise/news20050725/fitness-level-declines-dramatically-age

www.my.clevelandclinic.org

MENOPAUSE AND BEYOND

Fitness tips for menopause: Why fitness counts. (2021, March 12). https://mayoclinic.org. Retrieved September 17, 2022, from https://www.mayoclinic.org/healthy-lifestyle/womens-health/in-depth/fitness-tips-for-menopause/art-20044602

Lombardo, C. R. (2015, May 7). *Difference Between Menopause and Postmenopause.* HRF. Retrieved September 16, 2022, from https://healthresearchfunding.org/difference-between-menopause-and-postmenopause/

Mayo Clinic Staff. (2021a, June 17). *Healthy Lifestyle Fitness: Get the most from your workouts by knowing how to gauge your exercise intensity.* https://www.mayoclinic.org.

Mishra, N., Mishra, V.N., and Devanshi (Jul-Dec; 2011). 2(2): 51-56. *Exercise Beyond Menopause: Dos and Don'ts.* Retrieved September 16, 2022, from www.ncbinlm.nih.gov/pmc/articles/PMC3296386/

Pointer, K., & Wilson, D. R. (2017, April 27). *Move Over Menopause: 5 Reasons This is the Best Time to Exercise.* Health Line. www.healthline.com

Scaccia, A., & Wilson, D. R. (2019, March 7). *How Long Do Symptoms of Menopause Last?* Healthline.Com. www.healthline.com/health/meonpause/how-long-do-symptoms-of-menopause-last#noHeaderPrefixedContent

BONE HEALTH

Demontiero, O., Vidal, C., & Duque, G. (2012, April). *Aging and Bone Loss: New Insights for the Clinician*. Retrieved September 28, 2022, from https://www.ncbi.nlm.nih.gov>articles>PMC3383520

Dugdale, III, D., Sieve, D., Conaway, B., & A.D.A.M. editorial team. (2020, July 25). *Aging Changes in the Bones-Muscles-Joints*. MedlinePlus. Retrieved September 28, 2022, from https://www.medlineplus.gov/en cy/article/004015.htm

Falls and Fractures in Older Adults: Causes and Prevention. (n.d.). National Institute on Aging. Retrieved September 28, 2022, from https://www. nia.nih.gov/health/falls-and-fractures-older-adults-causes-and-preve ntion

Johns Hopkins University, The Johns Hopkins Hospital and Johns Hopkins Health System. (2022). *Osteoporosis: What You Need to Know as You Age*. https://www.hopkinsmedicine.org. Retrieved September 28, 2022, from https://www.hopkinsmedicine.org/health

Levine, H. (2021, March 16). How to Keep Your Bones Strong as You Age. *www.Webmd.Com*. Retrieved September 28, 2022, from https://w ww.webmd.com/healthy-aging/features/strong-bones

National Council for the Aging. (2022, May 12). *What Is Bone Density? A Practical Guide for Older Adults*. ncos.org. Retrieved September 28, 2022, from www.ncoa.org

National Institute on Aging. (2017, June 26). *Osteoporosis*. www.nia.nih.gov. Retrieved September 28, 2022, from https://www.nia.nih.gov/health/ osteoporosis

Robinson, K., & Zaremba, K. (2022, September 9). *The Top Anti-inflammatory Foods List: 13 Foods that Fight Inflammation.* https//www.fullscript.com. Retrieved September 28, 2022, from https://www.fullscript.com

Wartenberg, L., & Spritzer, F. (2021, December 10). *13 of the Most Anti-Inflammatory Foods You Can Eat.* https://www.healthline.com. Retrieved September 28, 2022, from https://www.healthline.com

DIET

Hughes, L. (2022, April 16). *How Does Too Much Sugar Affect Your Body?* WebMD. Retrieved September 17, 2022, from https://www.//webmed.com

Mayo Clinic Staff. (2021b, June 25). *DASH diet: Healthy eating to lower your blood pressure.* Mayo Clinic. Retrieved September 17, 2022, from https://www.//webmed.com

MyPlate/ U.S. Department of Agriculture. Retrieved September 17, 2022 https://www.myplate.gov

Sassos, S. (2020, October 29). *Everything you need to Know About the Different Types of Sugar.* Goodhousekeeping.Org. https://goodhousekeeping.com

U.S. News Staff. (2022, January 4). *U.S. News Best Diets: How We Rated 40 Eating Plans: With help from a panel of diet and nutrition experts, U.S. News unveils new 2022 diet rankings.* https://health.usnew.com/wellnes/food/articles.how-us-news-ranks-best-diets. Retrieved September 16, 2022 from https://health.usnew.com/wellness/food/articles.how-us-news-ra nks-best-d

Watson, S. (2021, July 20). *Dopamine: The Pathway to Pleasure.* Harvard.edu. Retrieved September 17, 2022, from https://https://www.// health.harvard.edu

WATER

Electrolyte Replacement: What to Drink, How Much and How Often? (2020, July). Adapted Nutrition. Retrieved September 17, 2022, from https://w ww.//adapted-nutrition.com

Fenestra Research Labs. (n.d.). *Clinical Research on Crystal Salt.* https://www.saltability.com. Retrieved September 17, 2022, from https://www.saltability.com

Ferreira, P. & Hendel, B (2003). *"Water and Salt: The Essence of Life".*

Fresher, T. (2016, January 13). *Pink Himalayan Sea Salt. The Perfect Electrolyte.* tanqva.com. Retrieved September 17, 2022, from https://w ww.//tanqva.com.au/post/pink-himalayan-sea-salt-the-perfect-elect rolyte

National Council On Aging. (2021, August 23). *Hydration for Older Adults: How to Stay Hydrated for Better Health.* ncoa.org. Retrieved September 17, 2022, from https://www.ncoa.org

WeMD Editorial Contributors (2021, March 23). *What to Know About Dehydration in Older Adults.* Retrieved September 17, 2022, from https://webmd.org

OBESITY

Crystal, G. (2022, August 23). *What is the Clinical Definition of Obesity* Retrieved September 17, 2022, from https://www.thehealthboard.com

Taubes, G. (2021, September 12). *How a 'fatally tragically flawed' paradigm has derailed the science of obesity.* www.statnews.com. Retrieved September 17, 2022, from https://www.statnews.com

Obesity Research. Division of General Internal Medicine. Retrieved September 17, 2022, from www.hopkinsmedicine.org

SLEEP

Leitner, S. (2022, February 24). *How Much Sleep Should I Get? Here's What Science Says.* saatva.com. Retrieved September 17, 2022, from https://www.saatva.com

Olson, E. (n.d.). *How Many Hours of Sleep Are Enough for Good Health?* https://www.mayoclinic.org. Retrieved September 17, 2022, from https://www.mayoclinic.org

Summer, J. (2022, April 15). *Eight Health Benefits of Sleep.* https://www.sleepfoundation.org. Retrieved September 17, 2022, from. https://www.sleepfoundation.org/how-sleep-works/benefits-of-sleep

Suni, E. (2022, August 29). *How Sleep Works.* https://www.sleepfoundation.org. Retrieved September 17, 2022, from https://www.sleepfoundation.org/how-sleep-works/benefits-of-sleep

FITNESS GUIDELINES FOR ADULTS/OLDER ADULTS

Centers for Disease Control and Prevention. *Physical Activity is Essential to Healthy Aging.* Retrieved September 17, 2022, from www.cdc.gov

Crystal, H. *(2022, May 7). How Your Health Care Needs to Change after 70.* Retrieved September 17, 2022, from *https://www.webmd.com.*

Easy Workouts For Beginners to Do at Home. (2022, March 25). Verywell Fit. Retrieved September 17, 2022, from https://www.verywellfit.com/ easy-workouts-for-beginners-3496020

MedlinePlus & Vorvick, L.J. (2021, May 3). *Exercise and Age.* Medline-Plus. Retrieved September 16, 2022, from https://medlineplus.gov/ ency/article/002080.htm

Tudor-Locke et al. (2011). *How Many Steps/Day are Enough?* http://ww w.ijbpa.org. Retrieved September 17, 2022, from http://www.ijbpa.or g/content/8/1/79

US Department of Health and Human Services. (2018). *Physical Activity Guidelines for Americans: 2nd edition.* https://www.health.gov. Retrieved September 17, 2022, from https://www.health.gov/paguidli nes

TARGET HEART RATE

Chamberlin, S. (2022b, July 27). *Maximum Heart Rate: Women are Not the Same as Men.* Catalyst 4 Fitness. Retrieved September 17, 2022, from https://catalyst4fitness.com/fitness-blog/maximum-heart-rate-women-not-men/

Measuring Peak Heart Rate in Women. (2022, March 25). Measuring Peak

Heart Rate in Women. Retrieved September 17, 2022, from https://w
ww.womenshealth.obgyn.msu.edu

Robergs, R., & Landwehr, R. (2002, April). *The surprising history of the
"HRmax=220-age" equation.* https://www.researchgate.net/publication/
237258265_The_surprising_history_of_the_HRmax220-age_equatio
n. Retrieved September 17, 2022, from https://www.researchgate.net/
publication/237258265_The_surprising_history_of_the_HRmax220
-age_equation

Martin, L. (September 16, 2021). "Rate of Perceived Exertion (RPE)".
https://www.medicalnewstoday.com/articles/rate-of-percieved-exer
tion-rpe-scalewhat-is-it-and-rate-of-perceived-exertionrpe#rpe-and
-heart-rate

Mayo Clinic Staff. (2021a, June 17). *Healthy Lifestyle Fitness: Get the
most from your workouts by knowing how to gauge your exercise intensity.*
Retrieved September 17, 2022, from https://www.mayoclinic.org.

Understanding Your Target Hart Rate. (n.d.). https://www.hopkinsmedic
ine.org. Retrieved September 17, 2022, from https://www.hopkinsme
dicine.org

Waehner, P. (2021, October 8). *Beginners Maximum Heart Rate Formula
for Women.* https://www.verywellfit.com. Retrieved September 17,
2022, from https://www.verywellfit.com

Williams, N. (2017, July 15). *The Borg Rating of Perceived Exertion (RPE)
scale.* https://academic.oup.com/occmed/article/67/5/404/3975235.
Retrieved September 17, 2022, from https://academic.oup.com/occm
ed/article/67/5/404/3975235

READY, SET, GO!

Cristol, H. (May 7, 2022). "How Your Health Care Needs to Change after 70". Retrieved September 17, 2022, from www./webmd.com

Frey, M. (2022, March 25). *How to Do a Beginner Workout at Home: A Step-By-Step Guide to Lose Weight and Boost Your Health.* Https://www.Verywellfit/Easy-workouts-for-beginners-3496020. Retrieved September 17, 2022, from https://www.verywellfit/easy-workouts-for-beginners-3496020

Mayo Clinic staff. (2021, March 12). *Women's Physical Activity: Regular Physical Activity is Crucial for Women Facing Menopause. Consider What Physical Activity Can Do for You. https://www.mayoclinic.org/healthy-lifestyle/womens-health/in-depth/fitness-tip.* Https:/www.mayoclinic.org. Retrieved September 17, 2022, from https://www.mayoclinic.org/healthy-lifestyle/womens-health/in-depth/fitness-tip

Mishra, N., Mishra, V.N., and Devanshi (Jul-Dec; 2011). 2(2): 51-56. *Exercise Beyond Menopause: Dos and Don'ts.* Retrieved September 16, 2022, from www.ncbinlm.nih.gov/pmc/articles/PMC3296386/

Tudor-Locke et al. (2011b). *How Many Steps/Days are Enough? For Adults?* http://www.ijbpa.org/content/8/1/79. Retrieved September 17, 2022, from http://www.ijbpa.org/content/8/1/79

MUSCLE SORENESS

Fetters, K. A. (2018, July 21). *Here's What Foam Rolling Is Actually Doing When It Hurts So Good.* https://www.self.com>Fitness>Goal Rolling. Retrieved September 17, 2022, from https://www.self.com

Hamer, A. (2019, August 1). *Lactic Acid Is Not What Causes Sore Muscles.* https://www.discovery.com. Retrieved September 17, 2022, from https://www.discovery.com

Rath, L. (2021, July 26). *Why Take an Epsom Salts Bath?* https://www.wedmd.com. Retrieved September 17, 2022, from https://www.wedmd.com

Samataro, B. R. (2022, March 6). *Sore Muscles? Don't Stop Exercising.* https://webmd.com. Retrieved September 17, 2022, from https://webmd.com

Santos-Longhurst, A. (2020, May 30). *23 Things to Know About Acute and Delayed Onset Muscle Soreness.* Healthline. Retrieved September 17, 2022, from https://www.healthline.com./health/fitness-exercise/23-things-to-know-about-acute-and-delayed-onset-muscle-soreness